Adrenal Reset Diet

Lose Weight Fast and Increase Energy with the Adrenal Reset Diet

KARA AIMER

ISBN: 1514375826
ISBN-13: 978-1514375822

CONTENTS

INTRODUCTION

We all want to live a happy and fulfilling life. But how can we live such a life when we have some deep-rooted health problems that mess us up from the inside out? Well, the truth is that life cannot be all-sweet when you have something that is harming you, whether you are aware of it or not. This is simply because the body will definitely signal you when something is wrong; it could do so through disturbed sleep, some funny habits like excessive urination, weird cravings, lack of energy and in many other ways. It is important to understand that every feeling you have is always linked to something within your body. If something is wrong, it will manifest through having undesirable feelings/symptoms.

The same case applies with adrenal fatigue; if you are constantly having sleeping problems, stress that seems not to go away, lack energy, wake up feeling tired, and have other problems like decreased sex drive, have allergies, asthma, dry skin, and a wide array of other symptoms, then you could be having adrenal fatigue. These seemingly nonfatal symptoms are likely to mess up your life and lead to lots of dissatisfaction.

But if you don't want that in your life, you can take action by following the strategies outlined in this book. This book will show you what adrenal fatigue is, how to tell if you have adrenal fatigue, show you the triggers of adrenal fatigue, the different risks that come with adrenal fatigue, as well as how to cure/fight the problem from its root.

WHAT ADRENAL FATIGUE IS AND ITS SYMPTOMS

Adrenal fatigue is a syndrome, which results when the adrenal function of your adrenal glands is below the required level. So, what are adrenal glands? Adrenal glands are part of your endocrine system and are positioned on top of each kidney. They are responsible for a whole lot of other functions related to hormones in your body thus when they get fatigued; they can affect your body greatly.

Adrenal fatigue usually shows as a combination of symptoms and signs, which can be at some point hard to figure out. Other names used to refer to adrenal fatigue include sub-clinical hypoadrenia, adrenal neurasthenia, neurasthenia, non-Addison's hypoadrenia, adrenal apathy, and adrenal exhaustion. Just to help you understand that this is not some condition from another planet, the truth is that adrenal fatigue has been approximated to affect up to 80% of people in the world, either for a short time or even as a chronic condition, at some point in life.

As earlier indicated, it can be hard to determine whether you have adrenal fatigue. To help you determine whether you have adrenal fatigue or not, let's take a look at some of the symptoms that are associated with adrenal fatigue.

3

SYMPTOMS OF ADRENAL FATIGUE

Some of the common symptoms that indicate you are suffering from adrenal fatigue include:

Difficulty waking up every morning
Insufficient sleep is one of the major causes of adrenal fatigue. Getting more sleep is one of the methods you can use to recover from this syndrome. Despite this, when you suffer from adrenal fatigue, you tend to wake up feeling 'foggy' and extremely tired even after sleeping for a long time.

Feeling fatigued during the day
When suffering from adrenal fatigue, your adrenal glands produce insufficient hormones that the body requires. This results to lower levels of cortisol and neurotransmitters like norepinephrine and adrenaline. Low levels of these hormones can cause you to have difficulties maintaining energy levels to keep you going throughout the day. However, you may experience a sudden spike of energy levels in your body in the evening.

Inability to handle Stress
If you suffer from adrenal fatigue, you will notice that most times you are unable to deal with emotional and physical stress. When you encounter stress, your body reacts by releasing hormones (adrenaline, cortisol, and norepinephrine), which increase your response to stress hence allowing you to increase your awareness, strength, and focus. However, when your adrenal glands get fatigued, they become unable to produce adequate

amounts of these hormones. Often you will experience a lack of apathy and enthusiasm. You may also show disinterest, anxiety, and high irritability.

Craving for salty foods

A part of your adrenal glands known as cortex produces aldosterone mineral corticoid, which works alongside the kidneys to regulate the way your body, excretes minerals and fluids. When the adrenal glands are fatigued, your body tends to produce lower levels of aldosterone thus you may excrete considerable amounts of minerals needed by your body through urine. You also tend to urinate frequently when you suffer from adrenal fatigue. Eventually, your body runs low on levels of essential minerals like magnesium, potassium, and sodium. Your body responds to low levels of these vital minerals by increasing the craving for foods that replace the minerals you lost. This is why you will notice that you crave salty snacks and foods, which may be a sign of adrenal fatigue.

Increased energy levels in the evenings

Low levels of energy caused by adrenal fatigue can make you feel very tired throughout the day. For a healthy person, cortisol levels reach their peak during the morning hours, and then decline gradually as the day goes. When you suffer from this syndrome, you may realize that you are suddenly feeling energetic in the evening or late afternoon. This is a sign of adrenal fatigue that shows in the earlier stages when your adrenal glands are still able to release significant amounts of adrenaline and cortisol.

A weak immune system

Cortisol has anti-inflammatory properties thus helps in the regulation of the immune system. In most cases, inflammation is an indicator that your body is fighting infections. Cortisol helps your body to prevent this reaction from getting out of control. This makes it important to maintain a balanced level of cortisol (not too high and not too low) for proper health. When your adrenal glands become fatigued, your cortisol levels rise thus the anti-inflammatory effect gets overly strong, which in turn alters the way your immune system works making it weaker. This state could last for the whole time your adrenals are fatigued hence you become more susceptible to infections and diseases. When your cortisol levels drop too low, your immune system tends to overreact to pathogens hence this can lead to chronic inflammation or even various autoimmune and respiratory diseases.

Other symptoms
Adrenal fatigue can also lead to other various symptoms such as dark circles under your eyes, dry skin, dizziness, weight gain, lower sex drive, numbness in your fingers, joint pain, low blood sugar, frequent urination, allergies, asthma, low blood pressure and loss of tone of muscles.

EFFECTS OF ADRENAL FATIGUE: WEIGHT GAIN

Do you know that you could actually be suffering from adrenal fatigue? It all begins with stress. When you constantly have high-stress levels, your adrenal glands have to continually release cortisol "the stress hormone" since your body senses that you are in danger. This puts a lot of pressure on your adrenal glands to produce cortisol. When you have high cortisol levels, your body goes stores extra glucose as fat in order to prepare your body to deal with the threat, which, in this case, is stress.

Once you know that you are experiencing adrenal fatigue, and its effects like weight gain, you would definitely want to know what caused it so that you can address the problem from its root cause. Let us look at various causes of adrenal fatigue.

CAUSES OF ADRENAL FATIGUE

Adrenal fatigue has been in existence but has peaked in the recent past as the world becomes more modernized. The increase in the occurrence of this disease can be attributed to the changes in lifestyle over time. As compared to earlier times, stress levels and level of toxins has been on the increase. Additionally, our diet has changed for the worse. In order to understand more about the changes in our lifestyle and the causes of adrenal fatigue, let us look at these causes closely.

Emotional stress

Stress is actually the main cause of adrenal fatigue. Each day, a number of stressors usually signal the adrenal glands to produce what we refer to as stress hormones like cortisol, which when produced in small blasts give us that burst of energy we need when we wake up in the morning and to keep us awake and focused. However, when we are constantly stressed and our adrenal glands have to continually release high levels of cortisol, the glands become impaired in their ability to respond and this is what leads to adrenal fatigue.

Inadequate sleep

So, why do you need to have an adequate sleep? Your body uses the time you are sleeping to repair itself. 7-8 hours (or even longer) is enough for the body to repair itself thus reducing the chances of suffering from adrenal fatigue disorder.

Pollutants and chemicals

Toxins in food, chemicals and drugs, pollutants in the air, antibiotics in the meat we eat, the chlorine in drinking water, pesticides in vegetables, birth control pills and many others can also cause adrenal fatigue. When these toxins enter your body, they alter the production of hormones by your adrenal glands thus causing a certain amount of stress on them. As you continue adding on more toxins to your body, the stress on the adrenals gets higher until finally they get totally exhausted.

Diet

Currently, we consume foods high in sugar and refined carbohydrates. Additionally, most people are too busy to prepare a decent meal so they just opt for fast food. Such foods trigger the body to produce insulin and cortisol to control the sugar levels. The more sugar you take, the more insulin and cortisol needs to be produced and the more the pressure on the adrenal glands to produce cortisol. This vicious cycle leads to adrenal fatigue.

Insufficient saturated fat and cholesterol in your diet

It sounds contradicting to what you have been reading about the negative effects of cholesterol and saturated fat to your health. Dietary cholesterol is actually needed by your body so that it can be able to produce hormones. Just don't overdo it.

Caffeine

Consuming too much caffeine can over stimulate you to the point that it forces your adrenals to work on the stress emanated by a caffeine buzz. Take a test of how your body responds to caffeine by stopping to take it for a while. The result will help you determine whether you adrenals are being exhausted because of caffeine.

Deficiency of zinc

Your adrenal glands require zinc to function appropriately. A number of things including grains that have not been prepared properly cause zinc deficiency. Vegetarianism can also be a contributor to low zinc levels in your body to some extent. You should consider eating foods rich in zinc such as soaked or sprouted grains and consuming clean & pastured meats.

Trauma

Adrenal fatigue is not only caused by long-term factors; extreme physical trauma may also result to fatigue of adrenal glands instantly. Earlier, it was said that one incident of physical trauma would not have any long-term effects other than just simple scars. New evidence shows that physical trauma does not only affect your health, but may also affect the balance of hormones in your body and the performance of your adrenals some time later. Examples of physical trauma include accidents such as car crashes and major surgery.

DIAGNOSIS OF ADRENAL FATIGUE

Sometimes it may be difficult to know whether you suffer from adrenal fatigue by simply relying on the symptoms hence it is critical to do a diagnosis. To diagnose for adrenal fatigue, you can either do it yourself or go to your doctor for a diagnosis. The doctor can run some blood tests and imaging. The blood tests will be used to measure the levels of sodium, glucose, potassium, adrenal hormones and pituitary hormones in your blood. Blood tests are done first; if signs of adrenal fatigue are detected, then your doctor might do some imaging tests. MRI's, ultrasound and X-rays can be used to show images of your pituitary and adrenal glands. A saliva test can also be taken which is said to be used to measure the level of hormones that are stressed. Some biochemical imbalances can also be detected using this test.

HOW TO DIAGNOSE YOURSELF

If you detect that you might be suffering from adrenal fatigue, you can take a simple test by yourself. This test is known as the iris contraction test, which is used to measure the stamina of your body in response to stimulation by light. If your stamina is decreased, then the test and your symptoms might be a clear indicator that your adrenals may be fatigued.

You only require a few things to run the test; they include a chair, a mirror, penlight or flashlight that is not too bright, a stopwatch and a dark room. Below is how to do the test.

1. Put your mirror in a dark room and stand in front of it for about fifteen seconds

2. Look straight into your mirror ensuring that you don't blink.

3. Using your small flashlight/penlight, point the light at eye level at the side of your head. Place it approximately 8 inches away to avoid damaging your eye.

4. Move the light slowly around the head to your nose maintaining the distance of 8 inches.

5. Once the light gets to about 45 degrees to your retina, stop. This is to avoid the light pointing directly to your eye, which can

cause damage.

6. Hold the light steadily then count how long your pupil can hold. Count up to 20 seconds. When your pupil starts 'pulsing' or stops contracting, end the test.

7. Repeat the procedure on your other eye.

Use the chart below to establish the level of damage to your adrenals.

Time (in seconds)	Level of damage to adrenals
0 - 4	Adrenal exhaustion
5 – 10	Adrenal fatigue
11 – 19	Adrenal dysfunction
20 or more	Adrenal function is optimal

.

NATURAL REMEDIES FOR ADRENAL FATIGUE

Your goal for treating adrenal fatigue is to restore the proper functionality of your adrenal glands. As you look for the appropriate treatment for adrenal fatigue, keep in mind that your adrenals are not the main cause of the problem. The best treatment approach would be to identify the root cause of the disorder. Depending on how severe your adrenal fatigue is, you may require different forms of treatment. However, common therapies and remedies exist for most stages of adrenal fatigue. The following are some of them.

Diet
To treat your adrenals, you need to follow a diet that will be able to reverse the damage is done and replenish them. Below is a diet to reset your adrenals.

Eat plenty of fresh veggies
Most people hardly eat vegetables and even at restaurants, you are likely to find many meat meals as opposed to a wide variety of vegetables. Vegetables are very important for your adrenal health since they provide a wide range of minerals, vitamins, fiber, flavonoids, and phytochemicals, which are essential for the repair

and revitalizing of your adrenals. They are also highly balancing and alkalizing foods. When you suffer from adrenal fatigue, you often have high acidity thus taking veggies will balance your body's pH levels. As you choose the vegetables to eat, focus on the cruciferous ones such as broccoli, Brussels sprouts, kale, and cauliflower.

Take at least a minimum of five servings daily of vegetables whereby one serving is equivalent to about half of a cup. Ensure you vary the way you cook different vegetables as the different nutrients are availed through various cooking methods but make sure that you do not overcook.

Eat fruit in moderation
Although fruits are good for your health, some of these fruits could actually increase your level of fatigue. Some fruits such as bananas are very high in sugar, which can lead to a spike in insulin levels and cortisol hence placing an extra strain on your adrenals. Consider fruits such as avocadoes rich in healthy fats and fiber since they can slow down the intake of glucose into your blood stream. Avoid eating fruits in the morning and instead take them in the evening or afternoon.

Some of the recommended fruits include mango, papaya, plums, pears, kiwi, apples, cherries, and grapes. Fruits that you should avoid during the healing of your adrenals include raisins, bananas, grapefruit, oranges, and dates.

Take quality protein
Consume foods high in protein to energize your body. Protein is quite suitable especially since it is quite filling and since it takes some time to be digested, you will not feel hungry too soon hence reduce the need to eat unhealthy foods. Protein also helps in metabolizing of fat and other important functions. Some of the amazing sources of protein include quinoa, brown rice, beans and legumes, liver, lean meat, fish, nuts chicken, shellfish, soy, and poultry among others. Ensure you avoid taking processed proteins such as processed cheeses and packed meats.

Increase intake of whole grains

Whole grains are high in fiber, minerals, vitamins and other essential nutrients that you need as opposed to refined grains that have been stripped of all essential nutrients. Consider taking whole grain such as quinoa, buckwheat, whole oats, wild rice, and brown rice. Keep away from kidney beans, as they are not digested easily. Instead, choose mongo beans, chickpea, adzuki, split peas, and lentils.

Eat some salt

I am sure you have been told how bad salt is for your health. However, when suffering from adrenal fatigue, salt is your best friend. How may you ask? Well, sodium is very important for adrenal function and usually when your adrenals are not functioning optimally, you usually have mineral deficiencies like sodium; hence, increasing your salt intake will help improve the functioning of your adrenal glands. However, as much as salt is important, ensure that you take Celtic Sea Salt instead of any other kind of salt.

Take more herbal teas

Since you are going to stop taking coffee and regular tea, you need to find a proper and healthy substitute. This is where herbal teas come in. Healthy herbal teas such as dandelion root have a wide array of benefits such as detoxification and healthy liver function. You can also take green tea as a substitute for coffee.

Take adequate water

Water is important for all functions including adrenal function. When suffering from adrenal fatigue, you may have the tendency to urinate frequently. You need to drink some water to replace the lost water through urination. Drinking water is something most people are unable to do consistently which can trigger a whole lot of other conditions. If you don't like the taste of water, just add some lemon and drink up. Try to drink at least 1.5 liters of water every day. When you wake up, take a big glass of water and you will find that you will be able to take some more as the day goes by. Ensure you stay away from tap water as it might contain toxic chemicals, which might add on more damage to your adrenals.

ADRENAL FATIGUE SUPER FOODS

So far, you have seen some of the foods you should get rid of to improve the functioning of the adrenal glands. Below are some amazing foods that you should include in your diet to improve adrenal function:

Bone broth

The bone broth has been used for centuries for healing purposes due to its nutritional value. Bone marrow is the main component of bone broth. It has been found to have anti-inflammatory properties, and can also help in boosting your immune system and in increasing the good cholesterol. Bone marrow also provides essential amino acids, minerals, and vitamins, which are essential for adequate functioning of the adrenal glands.

Seaweed

Seaweeds are high in phytonutrients and minerals, which are hard to find in your average diet. These nutrients are important in improving your adrenal function. You can mix the seaweed in salads.

Fermented drinks

Some fermented drinks are actually good for your immune system and for the enhancement of your digestive health. This does not necessarily refer to beer, as it is unhealthy for you. Fermented drinks are high in minerals and contain good bacteria, which can greatly improve nutrient absorption and digestion to release some load on your adrenals. Some examples of fermented drinks include kvass and kombucha.

ADRENAL RESET DIETING TIPS

Don't skip breakfast or any other meal: The most important meal of the day is breakfast. Make sure you don't skip it as it kick-starts metabolism and raises your blood sugar hence keeping you energized during the day. Taking breakfast also reduces the chances of eating unhealthy snacks such as highly processed foods that can put extra strain on your adrenal glands. Ensure you take your breakfast an hour after waking up.

Do not over eat: Overeating increases the load on your digestive system, which in turn demands more from your adrenals which make them more fatigued hence you feel tired.

Do no let yourself go overly hungry: Instead of waiting for your regular mealtime when you feel hungry, change your meal times so that you get to eat smaller meals at regular intervals. This is because when you suffer from adrenal fatigue, your body experiences difficulties storing energy hence regular meals are important to replenish your energy levels.

Eat a snack an hour before bed: Eat a healthy snack before you go to bed to energize your body as you sleep so that you don't wake up feeling all tired.

Make sure your meals have protein, fat, and carbs: This enables you to get all the nutrients you need to sufficient energy.

Add some healthy fats to your meals: As mentioned earlier, fats are good for you when suffering from adrenal fatigue. Therefore, make sure you take healthy fats such as coconut oil, butter, flaxseed oil and walnut oil.

Avoid white flours and white sugars: These carbohydrates demand a greater release of insulin and cortisol to manage the sugar levels. This adds more stress to your adrenal glands by making it more difficult for them to keep up with the demand for insulin and also stabilize the levels of your blood sugar. You can choose better alternatives for sugar such as raw honey, palm sugar, or xylitol.

Avoid intake of alcohol: Taking alcohol is not good for you when suffering from adrenal fatigue. This is because alcohol is broken down into simple sugars thus necessitating your body to release insulin and cortisol, which manages the sugar levels in the body. This extra stress on the adrenal glands makes the already worse situation worse. Therefore, if you want to get better, you need to avoid intake of alcohol. If not taking alcohol is too hard; you can start by reducing its intake with the goal of not taking alcohol completely, at one time.

As you change your diet, it is also important to avoid foods that you may be sensitive or allergic to. Food sensitivities and allergies may become delayed hence you may experience the symptoms a while later after eating the food. The delayed reactions stresses your adrenals greatly since it might read it as stress and result to production of cortisol as an emergency measure, and as we have seen, making your adrenal glands have to produce cortisol all the time puts a strain on them, which affects their functioning.

VITAMIN SUPPLEMENTS FOR BETTER ADRENAL FUNCTION

For the recovery of your adrenal glands, you can choose to use a wide variety of supplements. When you combine them in the right way alongside proper adjustments in your lifestyle and diet, you will move a step further in reversing your adrenal fatigue. Usually, when you suffer from adrenal fatigue, you tend to have a deficiency of a number of minerals and vitamins. Below are some of the vitamin supplements that you can use. The supplement needed varies from person to person depending on the deficiency.

Vitamins B6, B5, B12

These B vitamins are important as they play a major role in the metabolism of your cells. The improvement of your metabolic pathways is vital since it boosts the levels of energy in your body hence making it a great way to get rid of the fatigue experienced in this syndrome. Vitamin B5 stimulates the production of enzyme A, which plays a major role in cellular respiration. It also helps to break down protein, carbs, and fats. B6 on the other hand, helps in the creation of adrenal hormones. B12 helps in the repairing of cells, production of energy, and the maintenance of your red blood cells. The amounts required for each of these vitamins vary. For instance, to start with, you should get at least 100 mcg of vitamin B12, 50 mg of vitamin B6 and 1000mg of vitamin B5.

Vitamin C

Vitamin C is a powerful antioxidant, which is involved directly in the creation of cortisol by your adrenal glands. It also has a wide array of different health benefits such as protection from free radicals and improving your immune system. This vitamin is also a vital building block for proper recovery of your adrenals. You can start with 1000 mg then increase the dosage gradually over time. Liposomal or buffered vitamin C is the best form of this vitamin, which should be taken combined with bioflavonoids, as it would appear in nature.

Magnesium

Some studies undertaken have revealed that approximately 75% of all Americans have a deficiency in magnesium. Magnesium is a nutrient that assists in the maintenance of energy flow in your body. Low levels of magnesium in your body can result to depression and later adrenal fatigue. Other problems that may occur due to the deficiency of magnesium include stiffness, insomnia, and cramping of muscles. You should balance your intake of this nutrient supplement since taking in too much of it can also lead to problems in your digestion. Start at a lower dosage of about 400 mg.

Other Supplements That You May Consider

In addition to minerals and vitamins, your body needs a variety of other compounds to improve your energy levels and have a healthy metabolism. Below is a list of some of the supplements that you may use. They can be easily acquired from your local pharmacy.

Omega-3

Many people tend to have adequate levels of omega -6 but deficient levels of omega-3 fatty acids. This imbalance tends to lead to an increase in inflammation, which requires your adrenals to a step-up production of cortisol to deal with this problem. This weakens your adrenals further. Taking an omega-3 supplement can help return the balance thus easing the stress on your adrenals.

Acetyl-l-carnitine

This supplement is aimed primarily at boosting your energy levels and metabolism. It also helps in moving of fatty acids into mitochondria where they are needed by your body to produce energy.

COQ10

Your body needs this supplement for the production of energy needed to maintain and grow your cells. It also may increase endurance and enhance the time needed for recovery after workouts thus greatly reducing stress. Some food sources include; sardines, beef, and other organ meats. You can also use supplements instead of a food source.

D-Ribose

This supplement can help you maintain higher energy levels without stressing your adrenals. This supplement is obtained from sugar but doesn't mess with your blood sugar as opposed to other sweeteners and glucose.

PROBIOTICS

Scientific studies have proven the health benefits that can be offered by probiotics. Probiotics can help in the reduction of the side effects of antibiotics, improvement of digestion and may even lead to lowering of your stress levels. These properties are very important when suffering from adrenal fatigue.

By improving your digestion, probiotics help your digestive system to acquire more nutrients from the food you take. This allows your body to take in more of the vital minerals and vitamins that are needed to maintain your energy levels. They also help in the production of hormones needed by your body as well as support your immune system hence preventing regular illness, which can worsen adrenal fatigue.

It is recommended that you purchase probiotics that has about ten billion CFU's (colony forming units). The probiotics should also have at least five different strains of bacteria, most preferably Lactobacillus acidophilus.

HERBAL REMEDIES

Herbs are also very important in the recovery of your adrenals. They can be combined with supplements to improve healing. Herbs have been used for centuries for restoring energy and vitality. Below are some of the herbs that you can use to improve the functioning of adrenal glands.

Rhodiola Rosea

This herb is popularly used in Russia and Scandinavia. It can help in a number of conditions such as the poor circulation of blood, the tension of muscles, fatigue, and depression. By dealing with depression, you can manage stress levels hence no need for your adrenal glands to produce high levels of cortisol. Additionally, with improve circulation of blood, your adrenal glands can produce adequate amounts of cortisol.

Licorice root

This herb is also a great choice if you suffer from adrenal fatigue since it can be used to stimulate the production of hormones, increase your endurance and maintain healthy levels of energy. It also helps in proper circulation of cortisol for longer. The only downside to this precious herb is that it can raise your blood pressure. This is not usually a major problem since most of the people who suffer from adrenal fatigue experience low blood pressure.

Siberian ginseng

Russian athletes in the Olympics use this herb to improve

stamina. It also boosts energy levels in your body and increases your mental awareness. However, it can lead to rising of blood pressure hence if you suffer from hypertension, you should first seek your doctor's advice before using it.

Maca root

Research has shown that maca root has beneficial effects in the regulation of blood sugar and cortisol. It also allows your cells to take in more hormones much more efficiently hence increasing effectiveness. When you suffer from adrenal fatigue, you experience low levels of hormones, which can be corrected by using maca root for treatment.

Ashwagandha

This herb is also known as adaptogenic herb. It can regulate various systems in your body including maintaining a stable level of cortisol in your body – not too low and not too high.

CONCLUSION

The worst thing about adrenal fatigue is that you can even be suffering from it without even knowing. However, with the signs and symptoms indicated in this book as well as the diagnosis tests highlighted, you can know whether you are suffering from adrenal fatigue. Now you can know why you always feel tired even after a long night sleep. Once you identify that you have adrenal fatigue, the next thing is to correct the problem from its root cause.

As I have continually highlighted in this book, stress is the main cause of adrenal fatigue. Therefore, it is important that you find ways of managing stress like meditating, exercising, practicing yoga and deep breathing because once you can manage stress adequately, then you are halfway treating adrenal fatigue.

Thank you and good luck!

Kara Aimer

ADDITIONAL RESOURCES

Please point your web browser to **www.plaid-enterprises.com**
for more related resources, my full bibliography and to grab your
FREE book!

18267980R00022

Printed in Great Britain
by Amazon